The 90-Day Cardiac Recovery Plan

*A low-impact, drug-free program
to help you get your life back to normal
after cardiac bypass surgery*

The 90-Day Cardiac Recovery Plan

*A low-impact, drug-free program
to help you get your life back to normal
after cardiac bypass surgery*

By Bruce Huck

Author Impact Publishing
Woodburn, Oregon

ISBN-13: 978-1544841397

This book is not intended as a substitute for the medical advice of physicians. The reader should regularly consult a physician in matters relating to his or her health and particularly with respect to any symptoms that may require diagnosis or medical attention.

Author Impact Publishing
3326 Senecal Creek Dr.
Woodburn, Oregon 97071
(503) 765-6981
https://authorimpactpublishing.com

Dedication

To Karen, my wife—

Be not confused that you are not mentioned more often in *The 90-Day Cardiac Recovery Plan*. You were a larger part of my recovery than all the therapies, medications, and time that I invested in. You showed your dedication from the first day of the shocking news that I was having a quadruple bypass vacation—the fifth surgery that you have supported me through.

This one was bigger than all the other four combined. It was big enough that you did not have to do any sleeping on the floor. Your support then and now was invaluable. Without it I could not have had the success that the story in the book tells.

Thank you. Thank you. I hope for no more hospital vacations for either of us. But if life leads us that way, I know you will be by my side, as I will be for you.

I love you.

— Bruce Huck

Foreword

By Allen Knecht, DC

Bruce Huck is one of the most dedicated people I know. He "walks his talk" with regard to his personal health journey.

As one of his health-care providers, I have taken a functional medicine approach in my work with him. I had introduced him to Neuro Emotional Technique (NET), a very powerful stress reduction technique, and Quantum Neurology, a very powerful neurological rehabilitation technique.

When Bruce returned to my clinic after his open-heart surgery, I recommended my "Scars and Adhesions" homeopathic remedy formula to help speed up the external and internal healing of the physical scars. As is typical with this type of procedure, he had an upper rib severely displaced from its normal position. That resulted in severe rib cage pain with certain movements or when he breathed deeply, coughed, or sneezed.

In addition to manual mobilization to the ribcage and spine to reposition the rib, we also employed sensory nerve rehabilitation using the Quantum Neurology, Functional

Kinesio Taping, and Neuro Emotional Technique for the post-traumatic stress of the whole event.

He used the "Scars and Adhesions" protocol orally as well as misted topically over the visible scars. He also rubbed wheat germ oil (a very powerful source of vitamin E) into the scar twice daily. I have seen visible scars almost completely disappear with this protocol.

As I do with all my patients, I informed Bruce that I never promise a cure, but if I am successful in identifying the underlying imbalance causing a condition, that is when we see miracles. Bruce is a walking miracle, in no small part due to his unrelenting dedication to his personal health journey and to the mission he pursues in helping as many people as possible achieve optimal health.

I am blessed and honored that Bruce has crossed my path on this journey we all call LIFE!!

Contents

Introduction

By Kacy Borba Spann, ND, LAc

I met Bruce Huck in a networking group, where I walked alongside him as he grew his business, TriOasis, and as I began my practice of naturopathic and Chinese medicine. We were both traveling new territories as small business owners whose truest passion lay with helping others.

Bruce came to me for treatment and support for his type 2 diabetes. Our therapeutic relationship was a good fit. I firmly believe that each patient I see knows his or her own body better than I do. My role is to help them find their own path toward health and healing, as they define it. I often tell my patients, "It's your body, your choice." Bruce has been very comfortable with this autonomy and self-responsibility in his healing journey. He is the master of his own ship.

I am a dual practitioner, working with both Western and Eastern medicine. From Eastern medicine I listen to the radial pulses (thumb side of wrist) of both hands for certain diagnoses and treatment paths. It was because Bruce had been coming to see me for acupuncture that I found his intermittently irregular heart rhythm.

Like many Western practitioners, I have my medical assistant take vitals each visit, including the pulse. I generally take peripheral pulses (wrists and feet) only at initial visits or if a cardiac exam is necessary. This is the practice of many physicians in both mainstream and alternative medicine. I can't remember the last time I, as a patient, had my pulses felt by a non-acupuncturist, whether an MD or ND.

The art of medicine is often lost to technology, and not enough practitioners use their hands or solid physical examination in lieu of expensive, technology-driven labs and imaging. I am grateful to Bruce for reiterating this very basic and important lesson: Touch your patients!

It was his third visit with me, in February 2016, that I felt an irregularly irregular pulse, which prompted me to listen to his heart again. This time, unlike at his first two visits, I heard an irregular rhythm when I listened with a stethoscope.

I referred him to the Center for Natural Medicine for an EKG and treadmill stress test. His results indicated he needed further work-up, and I referred him on to Oregon Health & Science University (OHSU) and Dr. Albert Camacho, a cardiologist there. I would not see Bruce in my office again until after his quadruple bypass surgery.

Dr. Camacho was very kind and professional in his communications with me, a new, alternative-care physician. He recognized that our purpose together is patient care, and he treated me as a colleague and intelligent human. This has not been my typical experience when communicating with MDs and pharmacists. Often, the dogma of medicine overshadows the humanity of health care. Too many seem ruled by a scarcity mentality, as if there are not enough people in need nor appropriate roles for every type of practitioner.

We all need some of the many forms of care, and our needs may change with time as we age, grow, and mistreat our bodies, hearts, and minds. I am grateful to Dr. Camacho for his collegiality.

Bruce's cardiovascular dysfunction was caught early enough that he was diagnosed as needing a quadruple bypass surgery *before* having a heart attack. That early warning helped lead to a speedier recovery. At the same time, the numerous alternative health care practices he used in conjunction with the American Medical Association's standards of care contributed greatly to his recovery.

He returned to my office shortly after his surgery, and we got to work "surrounding the dragon." Surrounding the dragon is a needling technique in acupuncture that aids in the healing of scar tissue, allowing for better flow of qi (functional energy) and blood throughout the affected areas. Bruce asked me to take pictures of his treatments, because the number of acupuncture needles used with such large scars is impressive. You can see photos of the needles and the healing process on the TriOasis website (http://trioasis.com/scar-maintenance/).

Bruce's story is a testament to his intelligence and intuition. Throughout his journey, he has learned to listen to and trust his inner voice. It led him to question status-quo medical care when it did not work for him. He was also able to trust such care when it was deemed necessary and appropriate. It has been my pleasure to be a small part in his journey toward better health and longevity and to see his recovery with quality of life intact, if not improved.

Discovery

Prior Indications

It started with a regular appointment on February 3, 2016, with my naturopath, Dr. Kacy Borba Spann, of Beaverton, Oregon. We were doing acupuncture for my diabetes and some other health issues. She was taking my beats, as they do for acupuncture.

She noticed that my heart was skipping a beat. She was concerned about it and said we should find out what that means before we worked with other issues.

I had never had any indication of a heart problem. No pain in the heart, no pain in either arm, none of the usual signals of heart problems of any kind. Later, Dr. Albert Camacho, a cardiologist at Oregon Health & Science University, told me that it is common for diabetics not to feel the normal indicators of a heart attack in the making.

That skipped heart beat started my journey through quadruple bypass surgery and rehabilitation to a nearly complete recovery.

As I write this, it's been about six months from that first discovery to the time Dr. Camacho, my cardiologist, said I was free to check back in a year or as needed. My quadruple-bypass surgery took place on May 3, 2016. On August 31, I said goodbye to Dr. Camacho (unless there would be some unexpected need).

After the discovery of that missed beat, I went through testing and procedures approved by the American Medical Association. After the surgery, I thought there were better alternatives to the cardiac rehabilitation than those offered by OHSU Cardiac Rehabilitation. For my own rehabilitation and recovery, I used the same technologies I provide at TriOasis, my Cellular Energy Center in Portland, Oregon.

Through the five surgeries I've had in my lifetime, I've learned that when you have a medical crisis, there's no place you want to be more than the AMA-approved hospital. When you're done with that crisis, there's no place you want to be farther from than that hospital and Pharmageddon!

About TriOasis

I started my journey to what is now TriOasis in February of 2014. As a consultant helping diabetics manage their diet, I went to a similar practitioner in a nearby city to exchange shake formulas, nutrition concepts, and other ideas. I walked into that practitioner's place of business and found that the center used a hyperbaric chamber and LED light therapy.

I researched the hyperbaric chamber further and learned that it can regenerate capillaries in areas where tissues were stressed. The oxygen the chamber supplies can stimulate stressed tissues to return to optimum function, depending on how much the stress had reduced their ability to function.

That February, I began the journey that led to what is now my Cellular Energy Center, TriOasis. The following July, TriOasis opened, and we continue to evolve it to this day.

We opened with hyperbarics, LED lights, and whole-body vibration. We have since added hemp oil extract (CBD oils) and pulsed electromagnetic field therapies (PEMF) to care for the spectrum of pain, neuropathy, fibromyalgia, and other chronic and acute health issues.

We offer drug-free alternatives that can stimulate the body's cells as needed. As when you jump-start a battery, the cells that need assistance absorb what they require. Those that are fully operational ignore the stimulation.

The body's cells require three things in order to function optimally every day.

1. Fuel (which we aid with CBD oils)

2. Oxygen (which we aid with hyperbarics and whole-body vibration)

3. Electricity (which we aid with LED light therapy and pulsed electromagnetic field therapies)

We offer technologies to help provide cells with all three of those needs. TriOasis has become a full-spectrum center to help people with pain and other chronic or acute injuries and health issues.

Hyperbaric Chamber

Hyperbaric therapy involves breathing oxygen under pressure. Hyperbaric chambers have been used since ancient Greek days. It isn't something new or some phenomenon that just showed up. What is new is the ability to receive effective mild-hyperbarics away from the hospital environment.

Oxygen provides life for the body. We don't often think of oxygen's primary purpose, but food, drink, and oxygen are all part of the same process of helping the body function optimally. The hyperbaric chamber can produce incredible results by delivering 100-percent oxygen throughout the body. If you have doubts about the importance of oxygen, try to hold your breath for more than two minutes.

In the hyperbaric chamber, you go under increased air pressure and breathe from an oxygenator. The 100-percent oxygen is absorbed through your lungs into the plasma of your body. In this liquid state, oxygen can circulate throughout the body, except for tissue areas that have been damaged or stressed. For example, if you have an open-cut wound or maybe a back injury, the oxygen can generate new capillaries to feed oxygen to the damaged areas. Once it is fed oxygen that was previously denied, the stressed tissue can return to its optimal ability to function.

In my life as a diabetic, I have always worried about possible neuropathy, the lack of feeling away from the spine, especially in my feet and hands. By doing the hyperbarics regularly, I've increased the effectiveness of my body's circulation. The better your circulation works, the better your body can work. I'm sure it's a big part of what helped me avoid having a heart attack, as have many of the alternative techniques at TriOasis.

A recent study from Israel focused on patients who had had concussions. In the study, they used hyperbarics on the group. In this group were forty-eight people who had fibromyalgia, and all forty-eight of them saw their fibromyalgia completely disappear in the course of the study. It illustrates why medication, tragically, works so poorly for fibromyalgia. The conclusions need to be studied more, but the researchers concluded that probably seventy percent of fibromyalgia's pain and problems are generated from the brain.

With hyperbarics, the most important area that the oxygen gets to is the brain. Oxygen passes through the cell membrane easily. It can generate tremendous results for brain issues, such as in the post-concussion patients in the study. The use of hyperbarics needs to be studied more, but it opens the door to helping many people for many health issues.

As a diabetic, I could feel the difference mild-hyperbarics made right away. There was a difference in the clarity of my mind. There was also an improvement in my blood sugars.

At TriOasis, we can customize our hyperbaric sessions to the needs of the individual. Patients listen to what their body is telling them about what is happening, and we adjust the sessions by adding other alternatives the body may be asking for.

Most hyperbaric sessions last an hour. Many people are ready to get out at forty-five minutes, and some feel best when they stay in the chamber for ninety minutes. It's the greatest afternoon nap you'll ever experience.

Our hyperbaric chamber is like a small blimp. It's run with a compressor and an oxygenator. The compressor inflates the blimp and creates the pressure. It takes you to 1.3 times normal atmospheric pressure, which is like being ten or twelve feet underwater. Hospital chambers generally go to 2.2 times normal atmospheric pressure. You can get the same results over time, whether you're at 1.3 or 2.2.

Ours is a soft tank, roughly eight feet long, with a diameter of six feet. One to two people can fit comfortably inside. You may use the mask or go without it. Whether or not you use the mask makes a dramatic difference.

Using the mask makes the session six times stronger than going without it, because it directly feeds 100-percent oxygen into your body. The air we breathe every day is only 21 percent oxygen.

Some people can't wear a mask. In that case, they can use the hyperbaric chamber ambient—without the mask. The results without the mask will be the same over time, but it will take longer.

The idea of using the chamber can make some of our clients uncomfortable. Every day we get asked whether the hyperbaric chamber is a problem for people with claustrophobia.

I've had several people with claustrophobia use it. It takes a little more time to get used to it. We do some dry runs. I have that claustrophobic feeling, too, not severely, but I'm aware of it.

As the chamber inflates, it gets larger. You get the sensation that instead of being closed in, the space gets larger around you. Once under pressure, it's a large space. When I lie on my back I can barely touch the top with my arms extended. The chamber has multiple windows to see out of.

For someone who struggles with claustrophobia, we work up to a full session gently. Maybe the first time, the client just gets into the chamber, and we don't zip it up or pressurize it. The second time that client gets in it, we might zip it and pressurize it. Maybe he or she stays in the chamber for a half hour; maybe for 10 minutes. Just as with many of the alternatives at TriOasis, the experience is customized to the individual.

If they're in a crisis because of their health situation, if they've run out of AMA alternatives, the chamber is not that frightening compared to the option of staying in poor health.

Lights

The curative powers of light rays were defined by a French veterinary acupuncturist, Paul Nogier, in the 1950s-60s.

Based on his work with light therapy in France, race-horse owners brought the lights to the United States in 1972 because of the restrictions on drugs given to racehorses. The lights worked so well that the obvious next step was to use them for human beings.

At TriOasis, we use light pads imbedded with LED lights in one, two, or three colors: blue, red, and infrared. The light rays are absorbed by the tissue, generating the body's natural process to fight inflammation—vasodilation. The different colors penetrate to different depths of tissue.

Vasodilation is the body's ability to relax the muscles that control the pressure on tendons, nerves, and blood vessels, so that the interior diameter of those blood vessels can expand. When the vessel expands, blood flow increases. Increased blood flow reduces inflammation and allows for the relief of pain.

Lights can stimulate a more specific area than the mild-hyperbaric chamber does. The lights can be focused on a knee or an ankle, for example. The lights work on specific areas: surgery recovery, fibromyalgia, neuropathy, and feet issues. Light pads may be shaped to fit around the feet or hands. They work best when in direct contact with the skin.

There are seven different levels of lights, depending on the issues you want to care for. You might need to stimulate collagen during wound recovery. You might want more blood flow for pain relief. The controller has a timer that is set for twenty-minute cycles. We set the levels according to what your body has told you needs to be done, and the lights cycle automatically.

You can use the lights two or three times a day. You can come in once a day five times a week, or you can rent them for use in your own home. The schedule depends on an individual's needs and the time the person has to dedicate to it. A big factor in all of what we do is the amount of time our clients can invest in their own health.

I use lights every day. I use them at home and at TriOasis.

At TriOasis, our clients can use lights and the hyperbaric chamber simultaneously. It's a tremendous combination. We can do up to three pads in the chamber—back and shoulders. Using the lights in the chamber accelerates the effects through the body.

Whole Body Vibration

Whole-body vibration has been around since the 1800s. It came to prominence in the 1960s, when the Russian space program used whole-body vibration to keep their cosmonauts them from losing bone density and muscle mass while in space travel.

The machine is simply a plate you stand on that vibrates. It can go up and down or left and right, depending on the machine you are using.

Some machines, such as the ones we have at TriOasis, can do both directions at the same time. The up-and-down is a walking motion that engages ninety-seven percent of the muscular skeleton. The motion tells the brain that you are falling down, which activates muscles in an effort to keep the body upright.

To use the machine, all a person has to do is stand on the plate. We teach different stances or positions, similar to using various yoga positions, to focus on certain areas of the body or to avoid certain areas.

It's even possible to sit or lie on the machine instead of standing, depending on the person's needs. Whole-body vibration can be a complete body workout. It is the best core workout that I've ever experienced. The individual does no sweating; there are no gym clothes, no laundry, no need to shower. You can stand on the machine in your Sunday best and just do it.

When we were in training at Pro Vitae, what convinced me about whole-body vibration was watching a lady in her late eighties walk in from church and use the machine. She took off her Sunday hat and kicked off her shoes. She was in a beautiful white pantsuit with a gold necklace and other accessories. She stepped up onto the machine for fifteen minutes and went at it like a trooper. She stood on one leg, then on both legs, and stretched this way and that way. It showed me that this is the exercise of the new millennium. I've been very hard at it ever since, and it has changed my life.

Whole-body vibration absolutely changed my cardiac rehabilitation. I got out of the hospital on Saturday, and I did my first whole-body vibration session on Sunday, sitting, at a speed of 1. It was only at 1, but I was getting muscle stimulation weeks before the accepted recovery routine would have permitted it.

Pulsed Electromagnetic Field Therapy

Pulsed electromagnetic field therapy is the newest therapy we've added at TriOasis, and we're very excited about what it can do. Pulsed electromagnetic field therapy uses a mat, pillow, or wand to recharge the cells in your body that have lost all or part of their electric charge over time. The sessions stimulate the vasodilation process. Pulsed electromagnetic field therapy is a terrific add-on before doing a mild-hyperbaric session.

The human body is a large conglomeration of batteries, which are your cells. Pulsed electromagnetic field therapy charges the cells that need help and ignores the cells that are doing well. Like a battery, the cell will take on only the amount of electricity needed to make it viable again. It won't take on any extra.

Hemp Oils

For pain and other issues, we at TriOasis have added hemp oils, which are great for pain. We are discovering the benefits of cannabis without the THC. It's a product that people can use 24/7 without the dangers of THC and the problems it can cause.

Preparing for Surgery

Initial Testing

After Dr. Kacy noticed my missing heartbeats, she referred me for further testing.

I started at the Center for Natural Medicine, where I took an EKG.

I'll give you a hint. If possible, shave before you come in for an EKG, as they recommend. The dull clinic clippers can be brutal.

The EKG was abnormal and suggested myocardial ischemia—inadequate blood flow to the heart. I was sent back to the same clinic a week later to do a barbaric treadmill test.

The treadmill test consisted of a three-minute walk-to-running test on the treadmill at an accelerating speed. It's a very brutal way to approach this, but that's what the AMA does. The results on this test continued to suggest myocardial ischemia. They referred me to a cardiologist at OHSU.

Dr. Albert Camacho, the cardiologist who drew my case, had to miss our March appointment for personal reasons, so I went in early April.

He reviewed the tests I'd done and said, "I'm going to send you up to OHSU for a dye test on your heart. That will tell us exactly what's going on with your heart and the veins around it."

I went up to OHSU, and we did a nuclear perfusion stress test that was geared towards my age. I'm 64. I ran on the treadmill until I got up to 133 beats per minute, which was eighty-five percent of what they had predicted and wanted me to reach. At that point, I stepped off the treadmill and lay down on a bed. They injected radioactive dyes and took images of my heart after an hour.

What they found was a moderate-sized, mildly severe defect in the lower wall of my heart. They sent me back to Dr. Camacho.

Stents, Angioplasty, or . . . ?

Dr. Camacho scheduled me for another dye test. Five days later, I got a letter from OHSU confirming my next appointment. The letter said that I should plan to spend the night if they inserted stents and did other work on my heart. Dr. Camacho never told me anything about stents or angioplasty, but it turns out that this was what they were planning.

When I went up there on the 26th of April, the first nurse asked me, "Do you know why you're here?"

"Not really," I told her. "Nobody at OHSU is too good at actually telling you what's going on until after or just before the fact."

They explained that I would be sedated and rolled down to the operating room. They were going to inject dye into my heart. Then, depending on what it told them, they would insert stents, do angioplasty, or do nothing. They didn't know which course of action they'd take until the dye had circulated into my veins.

About an hour later, I was rolled into the OR. They told Karen, my wife, that it would be about two hours. She could go relax. There was a reader board in the waiting area, so Karen could follow my patient number. That way she would know what was going on and when I would be out. They told her they would come out after an hour and give her more information.

In forty minutes they came to her and told her that I wasn't going to have any stents, that I needed a four-way bypass.

Shortly after that, I was awake, and they gave me the news as well. Then we spent the rest of the day getting ready for my surgery. They were testing my veins, doing blood work, and doing whatever else they needed to do to prepare.

Later that afternoon, the head surgeon, Dr. Frederick Tibayan, came in to see me. He was the third one from the surgery team to come in and see me. He and the other members were wonderful. He explained to me the good and bad possible outcomes of the surgery and included all the cover-your-butt conversation that the surgeon has to include.

When he finally took a deep breath, I said, "Okay, when? I'm ready. Let's go."

"Well, I have a cancellation on the 3rd of May," he told me. That would be a week later.

We went home at three or four o'clock after being there since 7:30.

On the 3rd of May I would have a quadruple cardiac bypass.

Preparing for Surgery

I've been a diabetic for fourteen years. I've always had high cholesterol. It's a hereditary issue more than a dietary issue, and I had always expected that at some time in my life I was going to have to have stents or angioplasty or some type of the miraculous AMA work.

I work very diligently on my diabetes and my health. We offer several technologies at TriOasis that help the body function every day at its optimal best, beyond any type of medication:

- Whole-body vibration
- Mild-hyperbaric chamber
- LED lights
- CBD (hemp) oils
- Pulsed electromagnetic field therapy

I've been very diligent.

I see another doctor, Dr. Allen Knecht, a chiropractor who also works with TriOasis and our clients.

I had long been preparing for surgery every day, as part of my regular life. As it turns out, I ended up having a quadruple bypass without having had a heart attack. My diligence in taking care of my health is probably a big reason why I didn't have a heart attack.

As we headed home, Karen looked at me and said, "You seem a little bummed or whatever. Are you worried about the surgery?"

"I'm not worried about the surgery whatsoever," I told her. "It is not something that I can control."

I believed in the doctors and the nurses. I'm a very positive, optimistic person. If I were afraid of the surgery, I wouldn't go do it. I decided to make myself 110 percent ready for it and go in with that kind of mental attitude, with my body ready to deal with it. This would be my fifth surgery in my life—I'd had surgery twice for hernias, gotten pins in my right thumb and a plate in my right wrist. I am fortunate that all recoveries have been timely and successful.

On the other hand, my work at TriOasis is about inter-acting with people. I was thinking about the fact that the doctors had told me my work life would be shut down for 30 days. I would be out of work, in rehabilitation and recovery, for a total of several months.

I started making phone calls that afternoon. It's been my habit to attend multiple networking events every week—Tuesday, Wednesday, Thursday, and Friday. I also attend another four to six groups that meet once a month. Those activities are on top of working in the center six days a week and working at home. I was working six and a half days, roughly seventy hours, a week. That meant three twelve-hour days and one fourteen-hour day, with the rest abbreviated to what needed to be done. It's not an unusual working schedule for me when I'm fully involved in my job.

I was going to wake up after surgery one week later and find myself working zero hours and trying to keep TriOasis, my business that was less than a year old, going. It was a lot to think about.

Surgery

Checking In

When you go in for surgery at OHSU, they want you there at 5:30 a.m.

Going into the hospital was like entering the set of *Star Wars*. You go to the ninth floor, Admitting. As you walk through the hospital, there's very little going on. On the Admitting floor, however, there's just a buzz.

It's like being on a movie set in a space station, with people coming in and out. People coming to work, checking in patients for surgery.

It's a beautiful lobby area. Once you check in, you sit there until you're called. You're not aware of the outside world anymore. There aren't any windows. There are windows at OHSU, of course, but you aren't in contact with the outside world once you walk into Admitting and check in.

You write the check for your copay and then go upstairs and check in for surgery prep. You change into your hospital wardrobe and get comfortable on the bed to go to surgery. They will roll you out at 7:20.

We got up there probably at six o'clock. It didn't take long for me to change into my one-of-a-kind hospital gown and put my clothes in the bag with my phone and other belongings.

The prep procedure begins. A little more shaving this and shaving that. Then the anesthesiologist comes in, and you start that discussion. There were two anesthesiologists for the surgery. They put in the IV, and probably about a quarter to seven they started the first medication. We did chat about the fact that I was slow to wake up after my last two surgeries.

A couple of people from the surgery team came by, and it seemed as if everybody who is going to be part of the day checked in. At 7:15 they announced, "Okay, everybody, get ready. We're rolling out at 7:25." They ripped the curtain open at 7:25. I don't know how many people were there. It was like a Conestoga race to surgery. I was just about asleep. I remember the curtains being pulled. I remember Karen stepping back against the wall so she wouldn't get run over. I could just hear the commotion.

Waking Up

I don't remember anything after that until I woke up in the recovery room, where I remember a vision of blue uniforms scattering, which was probably just my vision clearing for the first time.

I do know that the breathing tube down my throat had been removed before I was awake, which I had specifically asked for. I didn't want to wake up gagging on that.

They rolled me into Intensive Care that afternoon. I don't remember it happening. I was a little fuzzy at that time. Essentially I was asleep.

Once again, they had a hard time waking me from surgery. They were a little concerned. I was pretty much out through the evening until about three in the morning, when the ribs in my back started to complain to me.

About three or four in the morning was the first time I remember being awake. The pain from the incision itself was never the issue, amazingly, but the effort to get to the fourth bypass behind my heart—as my surgeon explained to me—often creates issues with the ribs afterwards. It was customary to have pain from that.

It was a lot of pain. The process had also inflamed an injury in my back from many years ago. That made it worse for me than it would be normally. The pain woke me up and kept me awake.

First Day after Surgery

I was so thankful, Wednesday morning, when I got out of bed at six o'clock. The nurse came in to help me up. She was absolutely amazed at how well I could sit up—with her help. I was not allowed to sit up on my own. Once again, it shows why prepping to go in and working on your core muscles is so important.

And I stood up. Again, I did that better than she expected. Using the walker, I went over and sat in the chair. As soon as I sat down in the chair, the pain in my back stopped. It was just wonderful.

At 6:30 a.m., the kitchen opens for orders. The food at OHSU is terrific. It's like being on a cruise ship and ordering room service. They don't just say, "We bring breakfast at eight o'clock." They start taking calls at 6:30. You can order food any time you want. From morning to evening, breakfast, lunch, or dinner, they have a menu you can order from. Normally, aside from rush times, your order arrives in under twenty minutes, and the hot food is still hot.

My diet was restricted. As a diabetic, I never eat bananas, but I was concerned about having low blood sugar while in the hospital, so I ordered bananas and orange slices, regardless of the spikes in glucose they would produce.

I took thirty minutes to eat that banana and two orange slices. I was in no hurry. I didn't want to cough or get hiccups or anything like that, so I took my time eating. I didn't have anything else to do. I didn't want to watch TV the first day, so I ate slowly.

At eight o'clock, I went back to bed. They can store the food you don't eat in the refrigerator. You just put a lid or wrapper and your label on it. This allows you to have food at any time. You can eat good food anytime you want by just ordering and asking to have it put in the refrigerator. That's what I did. That's a big change in the hospital policy, and it is a wonderful thing. At the end of my stay, I learned that they record what you've eaten.

I told my nurse, "I want to eat again at eleven o'clock." I wanted to eat every two and a half to three hours at the most.

"Well, you can call," she told me.

I told her that I couldn't physically dial the phone yet.

I went back to sleep. When I woke up at 10:30, I got up, and the nurse said, "I've got your food here for eleven o'clock." She'd already ordered me another banana and orange slices, and I enjoyed every bite over another thirty-minute meal as I ate those.

Using the walker, I walked down the hallway and back. That's the goal they give you for walking—to the end of the hallway, which is probably a hundred feet, and back. Once again, the nurse was amazed that I could do that.

"I'll do it again when my wife comes," I told her. Karen worked nine to three during that week and planned on coming out to the hospital afterwards for the afternoon and early evening.

I went back to bed around noon.

I slept off and on. The pain in my back rib would wake me up. That was amazing considering how much OxyContin I was taking every two hours, but that's how bad the pain was.

I got up at 3:30 when Karen came. I walked again, and Karen walked with me. When we got back, the nurse said, "He walks really well."

Karen smiled at her. "He knows he has to walk to go home. If it meant he could go home tomorrow, he'd walk up and down there five times, no problem."

Then I went back to bed, and the greatest part of the day and my whole "bypass vacation" happened. A lady came in, a volunteer who plays the harp. "Hey, would you like to have music?" she asked. "You are awake and nobody else is!" We certainly didn't expect this. The lady sat there and played five songs on her harp. It wasn't a huge harp, but it sounded absolutely wonderful.

So Wednesday went very well. I was able to pee, which meant I was walking and pissing and only needed to be pooping before we could talk about going home. You have to do all three to even start the conversation about going home.

We ate dinner after that—Karen could order off the same menu as patients for only $10—and then I went back to sleep. They woke me up at 11:30 p.m. and told me they were rolling me from Intensive Care down to the Cardiac floor. Some doctor hadn't signed some form or whatever, so it took about an hour.

We got down there, and I had a great nurse the first night. All the nurses were great, even the overworked, grumpy ones.

The whole surgery team came to see me during the day. When one said he would be there at eleven, that's what time he or she arrived, not 2:30 or nine o'clock. I appreciated that they were timely.

Second Day after Surgery

At three o'clock in the morning, the nurse brought medication, and I finally got up and out of bed at 5:30 a.m. I had to get out of bed as early as I could because my back was still killing me when I lay down. I still had to use the walker to get over to the chair.

The chair was terrible. I'm lying in this bed, in a room that probably cost way more than $100,000 to furnish. But the chair literally has a two-foot pipe handle on the side that I had to use to manually lift the footrest, if I wanted to incline my feet. It was no Relax the Back recliner for sure. All this equipment that's worth hundreds of thousands of dollars, and I have a chair that seems like it came from a garage sale. It's an irony to me where the hospital feels it's important to spend their money—and where they do not.

The wonderful nurse went down the hallway and got me another chair.

This chair had the same lever concept, but it was comfortable when I sat in it. On the other hand, this chair provided the scariest moment during my stay. On Thursday night, I was sliding to the edge of the chair with the foot rest up to help lift me out of the chair. When I got my weight off the chair, the foot rest collapsed. I thought I was going to crash onto the floor. That was not a good mental image. Fortunately, I was able to slide just enough of my weight back onto the chair to keep me from crashing to the floor. I could feel my heart pumping hard. After that, I used the arms of the chair, not the footrest, to get up.

Escape from the Hospital

When Can I Go Home?

I was talking to one of the surgeons who came in to see me on Thursday. It was shortly after I had pooped, so I was physically qualified to end my vacation stay. I thought I would get to go home that weekend, even though I still had drains for my lungs in place. "When do I get to go home?" I asked.

She told me that in all the years she had practiced, she had only one patient who went home in three days.

"Well, I don't think I'm going home in three days after surgery, but I'd like to have the conversation now and not try to find somebody Saturday morning when I'm good and ready to go home."

She said, "Got it. That's good. You're doing great. Let's see how your lungs drain and whether you continue to improve."

The real problem was that my left lung wasn't enlarging and strengthening as it should, due to the pressure from the ribs.

Working toward Release

I developed a rhythm and a plan to get out of the hospital as soon as I was physically qualified.

I would stay up in the chair during the morning until about seven or eight o'clock and then get up and go back to bed. I would get up again around eleven or noon.

I worked on my walking; I made some firm decisions about what drugs are appropriate for me; and I focused on ending back pain that sometimes woke me up at night.

Walking

By the second time I got out of bed on Thursday, they told me I didn't have to use the walker anymore, because it just got in the way. I was walking the hallway around the Cardiac floor four to five times a day without the walker, staying next to the wall and using the handrail a little bit.

By Thursday afternoon, I walked around the floor. The nurse was supposed to have me walk three or four times a day. I would walk three, four, or five times a day if I could get someone to walk with me.

They told me that when Karen came on Thursday, I would be able to go outside on the observation deck. I could leave the floor, which I thought was amazing. My heart monitor, which reported to the nurse's station, was in place and worked remotely. Technology can be a wonderful thing. I felt very emotional at being in touch with the real world as we rolled through the door. I broke down in tears. It scared Karen until I explained it was just the pain and emotional exhaustion. I am an easy crier as well.

Drug Wars

By Wednesday afternoon we had finally finished the Lipitor battle. I don't take statin drugs.

That particular war had started as soon as the doctors learned that I wasn't going to do stents or angioplasty. Without consulting me, they ordered Lipitor for my cholesterol. The day when we were supposed to do stents, during the surgery prepping that afternoon, I got a phone call from Walgreens telling me that I had a new prescription.

"What is the prescription for?" I asked.

"It's for Lipitor," the pharmacist told me.

"You can cancel that," I said shortly. "I'm not going to take it."

The fellow of one of the head surgeons (a surgeon in training) came into the examining room the day we were prepping for surgery, and I told her, "I don't take Lipitor."

"You should reconsider," she said. "You have a long life to live."

"I don't take it because, one, I gain weight," I told her. "Two, it makes me more resistant to my insulin, and, three, it simply doesn't work for me. I've taken it in the past. It doesn't work for anyone in my family."

She gave me that incredulous AMA look and said, "Well, you really should reconsider and take it." I had had a similar conversation with an intern before, when we talked about what exercise works for a diabetic, versus exercising for the general public.

By Wednesday, the afternoon of my surgery, I'd had that conversation five times. Finally, they quit bringing me Lipitor, because I was not going take it.

It's part of fighting your battles in the hospital. Some you need to fight, and some you don't. You have to be your own advocate for things that do and don't work for you, because there isn't anybody to fight for you most of the time.

Back Pain

After we finished the drug war, Wednesday, the main issue was that my back was in such severe pain that I didn't feel safe going home. This is how people get addicted to pain medication. The AMA and Pharmageddon are better at masking the pain than resolving the cause.

My ribs and chest and the rest of me were feeling normal and fine. Not that I could feel much of anything with the OxyContin I was taking. But from what everybody was telling me, I was doing well.

On Friday morning after surgery, I skipped my morning dose of OxyContin so I could feel and figure out what was going on in with my ribs and my back.

As I sobered up, I realized that the surgery had inflamed an old injury in my back.

Shortly after I realized that, an aide came into my room. The aides usually just pick up the plastic gloves or clean up the bathroom. They're not medical people; they're there as volunteers.

I said, "Hey, young man, can you get me a heating pad?"

He was ecstatic that a patient had asked him to do something. "You really want me to get you something?"

"Yeah." I nodded. "I'd love to get a heating pad."

"Don't you worry about it. I'll get you one." He literally went running out of the room, and he came back with these little crack-open heating pads that last about twenty minutes. He handed it to me.

"I don't have the strength to open this," I told him. "You're going to have to do this."

He broke them open. I leaned forward in the bed, and he put them in place against my back. I leaned back. The heat melted the pain in my back like ice in the hot sun.

I had found the answer to dealing with the pain—not fixing it, but dealing with it.

I called the nurse and said, "Can I have my OxyContin now?"

She said, "You just made it. If you had called me twenty minutes later, we would have had to wait until the next session." She also was kind enough to order a regular plug-in heating pad. Sadly, I ended my vacation stay before it arrived.

I was able to take the OxyContin from the morning, and I continued with those heat pads every twenty minutes for the rest of the day. In fact, the second time I rang her, the nurse brought me about ten of them. "You don't have to ring me anymore," she said briskly. "I'll just come by every twenty minutes and crack them open and put them in place." For the rest of Friday, I used heat packs on my back. It calmed the pain so I could sleep a little. I was thankful to have found an alternative to drugs for dealing with it. Getting my ribs back in place became the major focus of my rehabilitation. That was something that was never mentioned during the cardiac rehabilitation process, nor was there any conversation about caring for scars.

It's another one of those experiences. Even though everybody knew I was in pain from my rib, nobody cared to slow down long enough to have a conversation about it, because it had nothing to do with my heart. That's part of my problem with the AMA style of medicine. Too many times the side effects of medication or procedures are discounted.

Parade of Experts

And then there was the parade of experts—nice people whose advice was one-size-fits-all. They also reminded me of the intern and his opinion on exercising.

OHSU gives you terrific pre-printed material. It tells about coming to the hospital and what to expect. There's a page of information about the dos and don't-don't-don'ts after surgery.

It's good information. But the non-nursing people simply don't do much educating.

The Dietitian

On Thursday afternoon I had my first visit with the non-nursing staff. The dietitian came in, a nice young girl. She handed me that sheet of general instructions I had already received.

She also gave me a couple of other pages from the Schnitzer Diabetes Center on taking care of your diabetes. The Schnitzer advice was a horse story in print. If I followed those guidelines, I'd be back on that table in five years.

The diet recommended foods like toast and bacon or eggs— daily. These are things that I haven't eaten for years and that no diabetic should eat regularly. It recommended them as part of an everyday diet. It wasn't merely amazing. It was shocking.

I wasn't looking for an argument with anybody who might delay my departure. "Thank you very much," I told her and put the paper in my bag with the other paperwork.

When I got the bill, I found out that the charge for her fifteen minutes was several hundred dollars.

The Physical Therapist

The next visit was from the physical therapist, again, a nice young lady.

She came in and gave me the same sheet of instructions I had already received twice.

We talked a little bit. "How are you feeling?" she asked. She didn't tell me anything about exercise or cardiac rehab or what I should do when I left the hospital. Nothing about that.

"Hey, why don't we take a walk?" I said, trying to get something productive from the visit. That way I could get a walk in without having to get the nurses to stop their day and walk with me. We did. We strolled around the floor.

As we finished, she slowly got in front of me, looked at me, and said, "Well, you're doing great. See you later." And she left. That was my education and activity with the physical therapist. Seems as if she could have talked some about doing cardio rehab?

When I got the bill, I found that the charges for her twenty minutes were double the dietician's.

The Occupational Therapists

There were two occupational therapists. Those two ladies came in, both nice people. One was obviously training with the other lady. They handed me the same sheet of dos and don'ts.

Again, there was no discussion of cardio rehab or anything I should do afterwards. They didn't ask, "What are you doing now?"

They did want to know if I was putting on and taking off my hospital socks. How they thought I could bend over or raise my leg to do that is a mystery to me. I said, "It is the pleasure of the nurses to do that for me."

I asked them to walk with me. Again, I was trying to get something productive from their visit. So we got up and walked. They wanted me to put on scrubs and got me scrubs for pants. The pants were deadly, because I could barely keep them up, and I was afraid of falling. When I was walking, most staff just put a second robe on my back, and away we would walk. But if pants were what the occupational therapists wanted me to wear, then that's what I wore.

Once again, as we finished going around the floor, they slowly got in front of me. They got to my door about ten seconds before I did, and they told me, "Well, you're doing great." And they were gone. But that's how they wanted to walk. They weren't really concerned about me but more about being late to the next appointment.

When I got the bill, I found that the charge for their time was double the physical therapist's.

Good-bye to the Experts

Those were my visits from people who, in theory, were supposed to help me. Combined, they were not with me an hour. The bill for their services was just under $1,200. Gee, you want to talk about the costs of medical care? There was no conversation at all about what to do when I left or even what I should be doing while I was there in the hospital, other than walking. I found their visits interesting. They were a part of that AMA profit center mentality that you really want to get far away from as quickly as possible.

Preparing to Leave the Hospital

On Friday morning, they took out the drain from my right lung. They said they would see on Saturday morning about my left lung. That doctor said he'd be back at nine Saturday morning, and, lo and behold, he was.

He popped that drain out Saturday morning and said I had to get an x-ray. "You should go home today." The x-ray got taken at 1:30. I got clearance to leave at 3:30, and I went home at four o'clock.

That was why I started the "going home" conversation on Wednesday. You do not want to be looking for clearance from the doctor who happens to have that weekend off. When you go into crisis, there's no place you want to be more than the AMA hospital. When you're done with that crisis, there's no place you want to be farther from than that AMA hospital.

It worked out great for me for the fifth time.

Recovery

Cardio Rehab

The following Tuesday, soon after I left the hospital, I got a call from a nice lady with OHSU Cardio Rehab. She said, "You have a lot of cardio rehab choices. We hope you will choose OHSU."

"What do I do if I come up there?" I asked her.

"I don't know," she told me. "But your insurance company will pay for it."

How can you turn that down?

"Let me think about that," I told her. I went to their website and looked it up. There was no information, other than that they offer cardio rehab. There were three sentences about cardio rehab on the website. Seemed to be almost as good as the other experts who had visited me in the hospital. Likely every bit as overpriced as well.

They did list a cardio support group on the website, so I decided to start by going to the meeting. I showed up on time and learned that it had been canceled several weeks earlier but had never been taken off the website. The only thing I went to didn't exist.

I got another call that went the same.

Then I got a letter from OHSU for cardio rehab. I'll call this lady, I decided. She'd surely know what she was talking about."

I called her and asked her what I'd be doing at OHSU Cardio Rehab.

"I think you come in twice a week," she said. They'll give you some exercises to strengthen your heart. You really should come. Your insurance company pays for it."

"How do I get there?" I asked her.

"Most people drive up here," she told me. Seems she might know I would not be driving. Maybe cardio rehab started about thirty days after surgery, not the week after?

"I'm not allowed to drive for thirty days," I told her patiently. "How am I going to get there?"

"You could take the Max or Uber, or you could take the bus," she said cheerfully. "There are lots of ways to get here. I hope you'll come."

The people who called weren't even aware that I wasn't able to drive.

I went to see Dr. Camacho after three weeks out of the hospital. We were having the meeting of "never having this happen again."

"It's interesting," I told him. "I can't get anybody to explain to me what goes on at OHSU cardio rehab."

He gave me that incredulous AMA look, expressing the disbelief doctors have when they discover that someone in the system can't explain something to you. By this time, I was used to seeing that look when I tried to get information about what was going to happen to me.

"Let me explain it to you. I'm the doctor." He told me to come three days a week and so on and so forth.

"Do you think I have time to come up there three days a week to do this?" I asked him.

I handed him my brochure for TriOasis and said, "This is what I'm doing."

My Cardio Rehab Regimen

I started my own cardio rehab the day I got out of the hospital, not thirty days later, when I could drive. I'll go through the things I did, and I still do many of them every day.

Air Foot Massage

I started doing Air Foot massage in fifteen-minute increments the day I got home from the hospital.

The Air Foot massage is a simple mechanical unit with an air pillow on top and a shiatsu massager on the bottom.

The Air Foot massage is important because all the major organs of the body are connected through the nerves and muscles at the bottom of the feet. The massage helps stimulate organs, muscles, and other parts of the body that had been through trauma with the surgery.

LED Lights

Along with the Air Foot massage, I used LED lights.

The light rays are absorbed beneath the skin and enhance and accelerate vasodilation. The absorption of light stimulates nitric oxide, which is a natural gas produced by the body and released within the body. The nitric oxide tells the muscles to relax. That allows the interior diameter of veins and capillaries to expand, increasing circulation. With increased circulation, you bring oxygen and nutrients to the tissues to help reduce inflammation and relieve pain throughout the body, allowing it to function better. Lights are terrific for accelerating recovery from surgeries, broken bones, and other issues.

LED lights have made a big contribution to the pace at which I've recovered, because getting the sternum and ribs to grow back together is the number-one issue of recovery in the first 30 days. The lights accelerate that process, along with relaxing and stimulating the muscles and other soft tissues. The lights come in pads of various sizes.

I use the face mask every day. It uses blue and red light, but no infrared because of the face. I also use a small pad we call a pain-buster on my chest, on the ribs in my back, and on my leg scars.

Exercise

I did simple exercises each day.

I started out with shoulder rolls. I tried to do about ten forward. I could do about five forward, five backwards, and then I would alternate directions back and forth until I could get up to ten in each direction. This is a simple exercise that stimulates the whole chest and all the other areas that were invaded by the surgery.

You can also do shoulder rolls while riding in a car.

I would do my ten shoulder rolls back and forth six or seven times a day, just periodically. This is like that first meal I had in recovery. There is no reason to hurry. In fact, the slower you do them, the better.

The other exercise I've done every day is walking.

Walking can be a challenge in the first couple of weeks, because of the lack of stamina.

For the first two weeks after surgery, I did my walking in my house. My house happens to be set up so that I can walk a big circle or a figure eight through the rooms between the front and the back of the house. It's nice and flat. There are plenty of places to sit down. I did most of my walking there for the first two weeks.

I would wake up at 2:30 in the morning, wide awake. I was suddenly between medications, even though I was only taking Tylenol at the time. I quit taking OxyContin before I left the hospital and haven't taken any since.

Due to my physical condition, my first goal was to walk for five minutes. After five minutes of walking steadily in figure eights or circles, I was fatigued to the point that I would go back to sleep.

I would wake up two, maybe three times during the night. I've never been a great sleeper. If I had trouble going back to sleep right away, I would get up and walk three to five minutes, building up to a longer walk each day. The exhaustion of simply walking would put me back to sleep.

Walking is one of the recommendations OHSU sends you home with. I felt much safer walking in the house for the first two weeks, and I could do more of it indoors. Walking thirty minutes a day in five-minute increments is every bit as effective as walking thirty minutes at one time. It seemed to be a better benefit because it would put me back to sleep.

The goal OHSU gives you is to work up to thirty to forty-five minutes of uninterrupted walking. On Memorial Day weekend, barely three weeks after surgery, we went to Lincoln City, on the Oregon coast. At the place we were staying, there were forty-three stairs from our room to the beach. On the last day we were there, I walked down the stairs, went down on the beach and returned to climb the forty-three stairs, uninterrupted.

I timed it from the top of the stairs to the beach and back to the top. I spent forty-five minutes in uninterrupted walking, and I wasn't breathing hard. Barely three weeks from surgery, I was up to their expectations of thirty-five to forty-five minutes. I didn't try to run or anything, just walked steadily on the sand, and took the stairs slowly, down and up.

That was my routine of cardio rehab.

Regimen

I bought a heating pad at Walgreens on the way home from the hospital.

Right away, I began a routine of using the heating pad, Air Foot massage, whole-body vibration, and LED lights the day after I got out of the hospital. I followed it morning and evening seven days a week.

The routine started when I got out of bed. At the time, I was waking up at 4:30 or five in the morning. I would go to the living room, sit down, and do my routine for forty minutes.

I started with a shoulder heating pad wrapped around my back and part of my chest. Then I reversed it for the second round. During the second round, I would put the heat pad on and place a face mask of lights on my back to work with my rib injury, which had become inflamed. When I used the heating pad in front, I could hang the small pain-buster light pad right over my sternum, where the scar tissue was.

I would run the heating pad for twenty minutes. The Air Foot massage runs for fifteen. Then I would move both light pads down onto the scar tissue on my legs and reverse the heating pad so the large portion was in front over my chest, the major part of the surgery. I would run that for another twenty-minute cycle.

After that, I would use whole-body vibration, sitting on a bench that fits on the plate. I would run the machine at the speed of 1 and sit there on a ten-minute cycle. I would run it at settings of 1, 2, or 3, varying it every few minutes. It's important to vary the speeds in the whole-body vibration, because the body gets lazy if you just leave it at one speed all the time.

This routine made up the major part of reaching into the internal damage of the surgery and accelerating the healing process, especially using the LED lights along with the whole-body vibration for stimulation and physical movement.

Massage

Massage was a big part of my recovery. I couldn't get a full-body, deep-tissue massage coming out of surgery or soon after. However, my masseur is a very good friend of mine, and he did come over on Monday, May 16, and did a whole session of cupping.

Cupping therapy dates back thousands of years to ancient Egyptian, Chinese, and Middle Eastern medicine. A therapist creates suction on the skin for a few minutes. Cupping helps with pain, inflammation, and blood flow. It is a type of deep-tissue massage. It has been great for relief with my ribs that were out of place.

Through cupping, he gave me great relief in the left part of my back, where the ribs were out. No heavy pressure with the hands. It was about a thirty-minute session, but it was tremendous.

Starting about three weeks from then, I have been getting my regular deep-tissue massage every other Friday with him. It's a ninety-minute massage. Since he's expert in different therapies, it's more than just simply a massage.

Scar Rehab

It is important to pay attention to how your surgery scars are healing.

After my surgery, I had large and painful scars where they cut open my chest and where they took saphenous veins from my legs to graft in as cardiac arteries. Today as I write this chapter, you can barely see or feel my chest scar. I've given less attention to my legs. Those scars are visible, but barely noticeable by feel.

Although OHSU gave me tremendous written material and in-person advice about going and coming from surgery, there was very little on caring for scars. Doctors looked at them in the hospital and at my early check ups, but other than "Keep it clean," they didn't say much.

I was told to be very careful with the wound in my sternum. No twisting, No lifting, No reaching out to pick something up. They believed that the sternum was most important, and I agree that it is important. But there was their typical lack of explanation of how they went about cracking me open or wiring me back together. I'm not sure I really wanted to know.

My Scar Rehab Regimen

I started rehab on my scar with my first day of physical rehab at home. Scar rehab was simply part of my program. I have had very little pain in any of the three scars.

Air Foot Massage

Using the Air Foot massage was part of the scar recovery. It may seem surprising to use the Air Foot massage for repairing scar tissue on my chest and legs. In fact, what the scars need is restored circulation. The Air Foot massage stimulates circulation in all the muscles that have been traumatized. The foot massage for fifteen minutes two or three times daily helped my scars as well.

LED Lights

The LED lights, while increasing vasodilation in deep tissue, also helped reduce inflammation and stimulated blood flow to my scars. The lights were were even more important for the scars than the Air Foot massage.

I used the lights twice daily, twenty minutes at a time, on all three scars.

It was while using the LED lights that I noticed that blood was pooling in places on all three scars. It was an ominous development that I would have to deal with.

Whole Body Vibration

Whole body vibration helped activate my chest muscles. It offered a low-impact way to strengthen my chest as the incision grew back together.

I started with the vibration on a setting of 1 and increased it gradually as my strength grew. It took a few weeks to get up to speeds of 3 to 5 and beyond.

Heating Pad

The heating pad helped my scars heal as well as reducing the pain in my back. It was an over-the-shoulder pad that I would use to cover my chest while doing the LED lights on my legs.

Cleansing

Although I was allowed to shower immediately after leaving OHSU, I was urged not to soak my chest or legs with hot streams of water. I protected the scars by keeping my back toward the shower head. Immediately after the shower, I would blow dry the scars.

Professional Care for the Scars

Both Dr. Kacy and Dr. Knecht gave good advice on how to care for the scar. Their advice was easy to carry out, and the results show that their techniques were efficient and effective.

Dr. Kacy suggested castor oil. I would take the jar and dab it onto the scar, letting it dribble down as I gently rubbed it in. It took only a small amount for each scar. I treated all three scars once or twice each day for the first 90 days after coming home.

Dr. Knecht suggested wheat germ oil. It came in small capsules that I would prick with a pin and then gently squeeze the oil onto the scar. I would do wheat germ oil first and then the castor oil, once or twice a day for the first 90 days after coming home. As my social activity and work picked up, I reduced the oils to once a day because they were getting on my shirts. This program kept the skin moist and allowed it to heal slowly and evenly.

My biggest concern as the scar healed was the pooling of blood.

As I applied the oils, I began to notice areas that were tender to the touch. I saw a little bit of pus when I pressed hard, and there was also pooling of blood. During a visit at the hospital and even before surgery at one of my routing visits, Dr. Kacy had warned me about this. She said she could treat it with acupuncture. I went in for my first treatment about three weeks after surgery.

I am a big believer in acupuncture. I have used it for my diabetes, areas of pain, sinus relief, and now for scar treatment. Acupuncture helped to restore the energy of blood flow in all three scarred areas. The improved flexibility and blood (energy) flow made my daily life better instantly.

At the first acupuncture, Dr. Kacy used 62 needles in my legs and chest. Visit my website to see photos before, during, and after the treatment (http://trioasis.com/scar-maintenance/).

Dr. Kacy did some puncture and cupping on the worst areas to remove pooling blood. I don't know how much blood she took out, but I do know that the relief was wonderful.

We did this every three weeks for six visits. She needed fewer needles every time. The areas of cupping changed as well. The worst spot was around the rib, centered over my heart, that was last to return to normal. That was the area of my highest pain, other than the nightmare in my back.

The acupuncture made an incredible difference in the re-hab of my scars, not just the blood flow for my heart and scars, but throughout my body to get the energy flowing optimally.

During this time, Dr. Knecht was maneuvering my ribs every two weeks. By the fall, the rib cage front and back had begun to feel normal.

Without the regular visits, I can imagine that my scar would be a bold statement on my chest and the same on my legs.

Thank goodness these professionals had a plan for me and my scars.

Daily Workout

From the beginning, I used the whole-body vibration, Air Foot massage, LED lights, shoulder rolls, and a heat pad. I did my routine at least twice a day, six or seven days a week, all the way through May, whenever we were home. When we went to the beach, I didn't take everything with me. At times, you do have to let the body rest, even though you're rebuilding.

Then I continued those regimens through June and July, not necessarily seven days a week, but at least four or five days a week—the same twenty-minute process once or twice a day. That's been the key to my recovery.

On the whole-body vibration machine, it took ten to twelve days before I could get off the bench and stand on the plate. Then it took a good three to four weeks before I could run it at a speed above 7 or 8. After five weeks, I was back to my regular routine. I spent five or six weeks at the P1 level, which is running at a speed of 35 to 60 on the machine.

By the end of May, I was starting to feel stronger. I'm still building my stamina. I went out to hit a couple golf balls in early August. I'm pretty well recovered from my surgery, in the sense that I can do things, but I'm not at full strength. I couldn't go play eighteen holes of golf, but I could hit a few golf balls or do different things.

Building stamina to be active is important at this time, but you also need to be careful about what you do. I'm not interested in starting a new problem with my heart. I'm just interested in continuing to rebuild my life so that I can live the way I used to and do it the best I can.

Social Recovery

I'm a big believer that you don't just go home and sit in the house. This is a problem too many people have.

I was fortunate that Karen could take the week off after surgery. We got up Sunday morning. Karen needed to go work and do some payroll. I got in the car and went with her. I didn't do anything at work but sit in the lobby chair, do some things on my phone and nap for the hour.

Then we stopped by to visit some friends who were having a get-together buffet for Mother's Day. We spent more than two hours there. All our friends were amazed to see me out. Five of them offered me a chair. I sat in that chair and never moved for two hours. The important thing was that we were out. I was out of the house.

My voice wasn't strong enough to talk above a whisper. I didn't do a lot of talking. It was the main reason I hadn't wanted a lot of visitors at the hospital. Talking was simply exhausting before my lungs had done most of their recovery. I told a few of my favorite anecdotes about the nurses, but other than that, I just sat and listened. I was out of the house and seeing other people, which is important in rehab.

You have to be careful. I wasn't doing anything physical. I didn't pour water. I didn't dish up any fruit. It was all done for me, but at least I was out and able to listen and talk to people.

On Monday afternoon, we went over to Starbucks and had a beverage. It was a beautiful sunny day.

We sat out on the porch. I put pictures of it on Facebook.

Tuesday was pretty much at home.

Wednesday, Karen had to go to work in the morning. I go to a regular networking event downtown on Wednesday mornings. She dropped me off for the last twenty minutes of it. A friend of mine who's part of the group took me to her office, which is close to Karen's work. I just hung out there, sat in a chair, and talked to her and joked around through noon. Karen picked me up and I went home and went to sleep.

I started networking a week and a day after surgery, going back and seeing some friends.

In the first thirty days of rehab, it was common for me to sleep thirty minutes in the morning and an hour to an hour and a half in the afternoon every day. It wasn't anything I was going to fight. You get exhausted quickly after surgery. Sleep is very important to the recovery process for the body.

I didn't ask many people to visit, and I discouraged people from visiting in those first thirty days, because carrying on a conversion longer than a minute or two was very difficult then. My lungs were still building strength. I talked in a loud whisper most of the time. Talking was also very exhausting, so the naps were important.

Getting out is an important part of rehab, but you have to be cautious. I didn't go anyplace where I would have to walk a long way. I didn't lift anything, even to pour a glass of water. Everybody did things for me. Everybody was very generous.

It's a big part of the recovery process to have social activity beyond visitors at your home. An even bigger help was that Karen's staff brought us dinner for three weeks. It was interesting to eat the different favorite family meals that were so wonderfully prepared.

The following Wednesday, I did return to TriOasis from nine to noon. Karen drove me there, and Uber drove me home. The following week, which would be Tuesday the 16th, I returned to TriOasis and worked from nine to noon or nine to one, Tuesday, Wednesday, and Thursday. Karen would drive me to work on her way to work, and then I would get Uber or my friend Cosmo to drive me home.

That was my start back to work. Two weeks after surgery, I started showing up at some of my networking groups as well.

I went to my first networking event the Wednesday after surgery. I went back to TriOasis the second Wednesday after surgery. I started to regularly go to TriOasis three weeks after surgery. But I was only mentally, not physically engaged in working two to five hours a day, three or four days a week. TriOasis wasn't open on Fridays or Saturdays through the month of May.

I worked with the clients who could make it in on that schedule. It was important to show them that I was doing well after the surgery and gaining strength. My clients needed to trust that the business would stay alive, that I would be there to help them. I slowly built up to three to six hours a day, four to five days a week.

I was working again, but it was even more important that I was busy and out sharing human conversation.

I'm fortunate that my work doesn't involve digging ditches or picking up fifty pounds or anything like that. When I went back to work, I was just talking to people, being out in public, and not sitting at home.

At TriOasis I could do my lights and the rest of my routine three times a day. I would take a nap and do lights and my Air Foot massage right at the center. I was increasing my rehab work while also returning to work, being active, and having social contact.

I continued with that through May, adding back my four regular network activities that I do each month.

Of course, I couldn't drive immediately after surgery. The last weekend of May, when we went to the beach, I did a little driving. There were areas of the highway that were very straight, that didn't involve turning the wheel a lot. I could drive in those areas. I started driving my own car 30 days after surgery.

You don't realize how exhausting driving a car is until you've had a quadruple bypass and then start driving again. It's mentally exhausting and physically exhausting because of the need to move your chest. It's important to plan where you're going and make sure you can get there and back. Then you need to rest. There's no way you're driving three hours or anything like that.

You have to make a slow, steady increase in activity where it's safe. You don't want to do any of these activities to exhaustion. You just do them to your level of ability, and then you make sure you get your naps and rest in between.

Speedy Recovery

A little over two months after surgery, Dr. Knecht told me that in his twenty years of practice, he had never seen anyone recover faster from a quadruple bypass. Preparation is a big part of it. My preparation was deliberate. Even though I did not know that the surgery was coming, I was ready for it anyway.

When Dr. Knecht checked out my heart, his testing showed that all the chambers and other functions of my heart are working perfectly. He had no doubts about anything. I haven't had any experience that leads me to think anything different.

Other Professionals

I have continued to work with my acupuncturist and my chiropractor. I didn't do any physical therapy or anything, but I intended to check in with the cardiologist three weeks after surgery.

I first went to my chiropractor, Dr. Allen Knecht, on the 11th of May, just barely a week after surgery. I was still in so much pain from my ribs that I couldn't do much.

With his genius and tools, he was able to do some gentle work on my ribs in front, working around the surgery, and doing a little on my back. He gave me a great deal of relief in my back. I would continue to see him every other week, and still do, and we've got it down to where there's just one rib in the front of my rib cage that is still bothering me. The rest have been worked back into normal position.

Acupuncture has been really important. Dr. Kacy, who discovered that my heart was not beating correctly, visited me at the hospital and informed me we would be doing acupuncture in the scar tissue area, both where they harvested veins from my legs and where they had accessed my heart.

My first appointment with Dr. Kacy was on June 6. I went to see her every three weeks. Today, if you didn't know I'd had cardiac surgery, you could not tell it by the scar tissue on my chest unless you were looking hard for it. Between Dr. Knecht, with his wheat oil and other help with the skin care, and the castor oil from Dr. Kacy, the recovery has been amazing. That process will go on for the rest of the year. At the end, my scar will be virtually gone.

From before to after Surgery

By August I was working six days a week with one twelve-hour day at most. Most of my workdays are six to seven hours long. I might take a nap, usually on Friday afternoons.

I take rest periods, but don't go to sleep the way I would in the early days.

There were days in the early months after surgery, Thursdays and Fridays usually, that my body simply told me, "I've had enough." I can lock the door at work when I'm done with clients. I just lie on the recliner and go to sleep. I don't have to worry about working through fatigue or exhaustion. If I feel it coming—and it's obvious that it's coming; nothing is unexpected—I'm allowed to just go off and go to sleep. I don't have to worry about it. I can rest. I can work freely, but at the same time I know that if my body hits that wall, hits that exhaustion, I don't have any problem with lying down and going to sleep.

Three months after surgery, I was working at about sixty to seventy percent of my pre-surgery schedule. I'm not in a giant hurry to make it more than that. I may work at only seventy to seventy-five percent of my previous hours forever. TriOasis is now well over a year old. A lot of the pre-marketing is done. I'm getting other people involved, now that we have something to promote and market, so I can do less of that and just be at the center helping people.

Before surgery, my weeks were commonly seventy hours or more, and now I'm working forty, maybe fifty hours. I have much shorter days, and much more rest during the day than I did before. I will continue with that schedule until my body says, "You can do more." It's all about being smart.

There's nothing smart about overly testing my heart. My physical health has improved overall. I had a lump in my left shoulder since high school from automobile accidents, pinched nerves, skimobile. The trouble was always in my left shoulder.

I've had thousands of dollars of rehab, acupuncture, massage, and electrotherapy. The lump would get better but never go away. When I woke up from surgery and got sober from the OxyContin, the lump in my left shoulder was gone. Nobody has an explanation, but I am sure it's that injury that began the clot that clogged my veins. I had one vein that was completely clogged and three that were impaired. I am sure the one that was completely clogged was affected by this beating my left shoulder has taken over the years. Now the problem is completely gone.

The disappearance of that lump reduced the daily pain I experienced by probably the last ten percent. I live virtually without pain today, compared to what I had before surgery. Surgery wasn't ever suggested as a cure for this problem with my shoulder. But it's nice to have a positive side effect from the surgery.

I am finding things out as I gain strength, build my stamina, and return to my daily life. I can now lift fifty or sixty pounds without being worried by it. Could I do it fifty times in a row? I'm not going to try that, but I know I can lift it.

The only activity that makes me breathe hard or gasp is bending over. It doesn't matter how much weight I'm holding. It's like the rush of standing up with something, walking with it, and setting it back down. I can feel my heart change speeds. I'm sure it's just exertion by the whole body as I bend. But my walking, my stamina, and my everyday life seem to be pretty normal.

As I write this, I have an appointment to see Dr. Camacho on the 31st of August. They will test my heart four months out from surgery. They're going to do the dye test and some other things, probably including one of those barbaric treadmill tests. They'll test my heart to see how it is in relation to how they expect it to be. That will be an interesting day.

I think surgery has brought improvements in my health besides repairing my heart. That was not part of any plan, but it happened. Some of these other processes and procedures that both Dr. Kacy and Dr. Knecht had me working on will work even better now.

I hope my diabetes will become a type 2 instead of becoming a type 1, as it was three years ago. We'll find out.

Nothing will make you pay attention to your heart like bypass surgery. Puts you right on top of it.

I have one rib that still gives me a lot of trouble. I think once we finally get that in, hopefully in the next month, I'll feel my heart less than I do now. But I'm sure I'll always be very much aware of it.

Looking toward the Future

See You in a Year!

As I went to bed on August 30, I began to feel the nervous energy of completing my three-plus months of cardio rehab through TriOasis.

Not the OHSU program, which no one on the phone could explain to me. They could only say, "You should come. Your insurance will pay for it." It was the same with my insurance company! They could not explain what the program was, but they assured me they were glad to pay for it. Sadly, they do not pay TriOasis to do rehab.

I woke up at 3 a.m. on August 30 and felt the déjà vu of waking up in an intensive care unit at the same time on May 3. I was alone in a dark room, lying in the bedroom wondering about my heart. The big difference was that I could get out of bed myself and go back to sleep, because I finally had the pain from my ribs under control. Not completely pain free, but the pain was reduced so that I could sleep without my ribs waking me, as they had done every few hours starting with that 3 a.m. wake-up in intensive care.

My appointment that August morning was the echo and dye test at 8:15. Then I went to see Dr. Camacho at 10:15. Allie was terrific with the test. The echo had some scary moments, as he found points of my ribs that were still tender to the heavy touch that the echo gram requires. The dye test had no such pain, except for the minor poke to insert the catheter for the dye to be inserted. The tests were completed, and I was in the waiting room by 9 a.m.

I was escorted to a room at 10 a.m., and Dr. Camacho came in at 10:15. He proceeded with the routine exam with his stethoscope, questions, and reviewing the test results. Then came the news.

As with the first visit thirty days after surgery, I had tested out above normal with my recovery. There was no need to change my medications. He gave his approval for me to continue with the hemp oil for sleeping and for what little pain I was having. At every appointment, I tested above normal.

I encouraged him to come by TriOasis and see the new millennium of cardio rehab, so he could discover firsthand why I was doing so well. He did take a few moments to look at the brochure I brought him, so he could see what I was doing for my cardio rehab. Then he said he would see me in a year unless some complication came up that I felt he should see me about. We closed with the weight control conversation and living healthfully for many years to come. He started with the comment, "All this you probably know."

He was right. I do. I told him, "If you can come up with a positive weight-control or weight-loss program for those of us who are insulin resistant, I am ready to use it." The simple plan he explained, like portion control and exercise, is not the answer for the millions who suffer from being insulin resistant. We produce enough insulin, but our body does not use it well. That excess puts the body mentally into fat storage, even with portion control and exercise!

We closed with his releasing me, and everyone agreeing that it was wonderful to see the results of doing cardio rehab at TriOasis versus cardio rehab at OHSU.

Preparing for Life Beyond Surgery

I'm fourteen years a diabetic. I've been through that journey, trying to reduce the pain levels that I live with.

Today, I live in zero percent of the pain that I lived in every day fourteen years ago. This releasing of my shoulder that for whatever reason came about through the heart surgery is the last part.

My right ankle has also been damaged. Being a basketball junkie, I was on crutches three times in my life. (Well, I am an NBA junkie, too.)

I have areas of my body that have been extremely beat up, and so I'm very aware of what I've gone through in the process of trying to reduce the pain without drugs for myself. Those positive results I've had with that is what I try to share with people through TriOasis.

I've become aware of what's happening in my body, especially as a layman. I run a Cellular Energy Center for relieving pain. TriOasis can help a lot of people with their health, but I'm not a medical doctor. I can diagnose for myself, but I'm not allowed to diagnose for other people. Without diagnosing for them, I try to give them a pathway through which their body can speak to them about the direction to take. They have to take responsibility for doing it. The alternatives that TriOasis offers are drug free. At the beginning and middle of the journey, these alternatives may hurt worse than standard medical care, because of the transitioning process of the body.

I have serious conversations with my chiropractor, acupuncturist, and my naturopathic doctor. I am not a passive patient of these wonderful people, who were brilliant enough to recognize that I needed help with my heart and got me there before I had a heart attack. But my philosophy doesn't deal with crisis, like the AMA does. We leave the crisis to the AMA, because there's nobody better than that.

When you're in for surgery or other crisis treatment, it's you against the hospital. You need to be well informed before you get onto that surgery table and into that hospital bed.

It's not just about physically preparing for your rehab. You need to be informed about what's going to happen, whatever number of days you're there, so that you can do the best you can. It's not about being in a fight, but you need to be aware of the philosophies of the people who are helping you. The AMA philosophy and my philosophy are very different.

TriOasis has a lot to offer that can help people avoid crisis treatment and survive past it. We can help people understand and make sound and healthy decisions. Doctor Knecht told me he's never seen anybody recover as fast or as well from a quadruple bypass. We both agreed that it was because I am on top of it. I try things and do way more than the average person would do in the search for the answers both to my diabetes and to reduce the pain.

It has proved positive for me, and I hope it will help redefine living normally for many people in the future.